All about your CD...

Please listen to this CD! It has magical powers as it brings our Clickety characters to life.

Butters the Fluttery Butterfly and Nat the Chatty Bat are introduced by the very talented Catherine Tate. She reads the stories in her own special way! You will laugh a lot!

This CD is another way to enjoy this book. You can listen to it in the car or at home or even at school. Try reading the book along with Catherine Tate or let a grown-up point at the words.

Listen to all of the UTT and AT words in these stories. There are LOADS of them.

At the end of each story on the CD, there is a little game. If you would like to join in, that would be great!

We hope you have lots of fun.

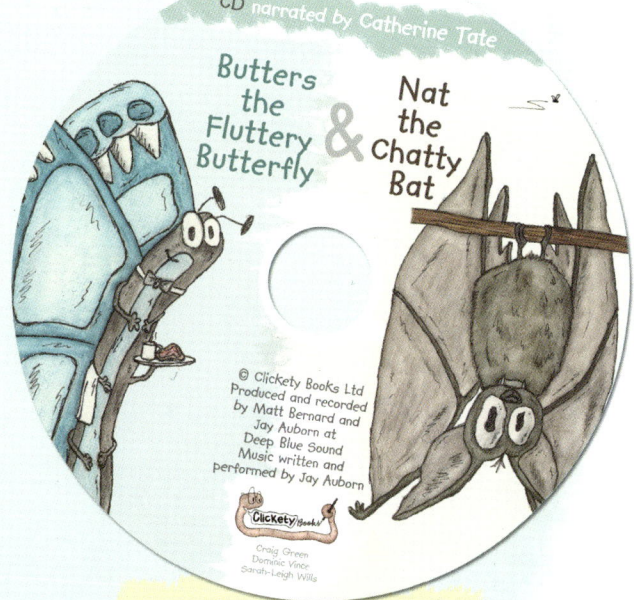

CD narrated by Catherine Tate

Butters the Fluttery Butterfly & Nat the Chatty Bat

© Clickety Books Ltd
Produced and recorded by Matt Bernard and Jay Auborn at Deep Blue Sound
Music written and performed by Jay Auborn

Clickety Books

Craig Green
Dominic Vince
Sarah-Leigh Wills

*You can find this CD in the back of this book!

Visit www.clicketybooks.co.uk for lots of fun activities.

D1795080

Special thanks to the amazing Clickety team

To David and Diana, aka Mum and Dad.
Thank you for your endless patience and belief.
Much love - CG

To Peter - DV

For my beloved Michael – SLW

First published in 2012 by Clickety Books Ltd
Tremough Innovation Centre
Penryn TR10 9TA

Reprinted 2013

Created by Craig Green

Written by Craig Green and Dominic Vince
Illustrated by Sarah-Leigh Wills

Speech and Language Therapy advisor
Sally Bates PhD, CertMRCSLT, FHEA

Series editor
Anne Ayre BSc, CertMRCSLT, MASLTIP

CD narrated by Catherine Tate

www.clicketybooks.co.uk

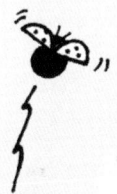

Contents

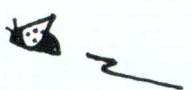

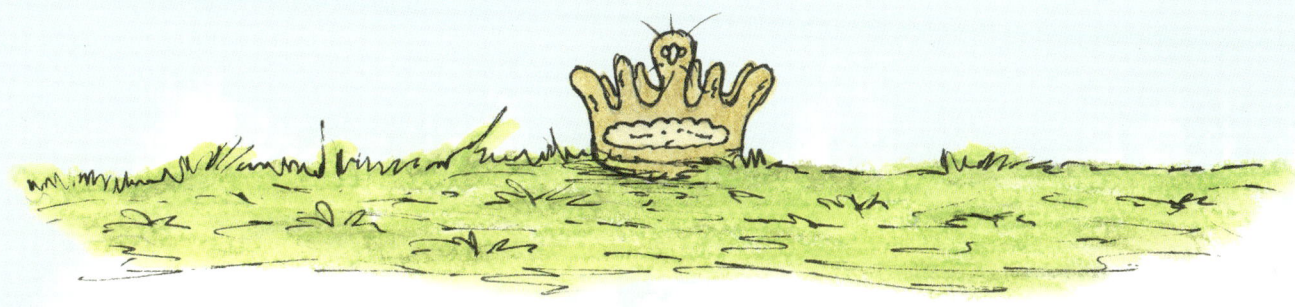

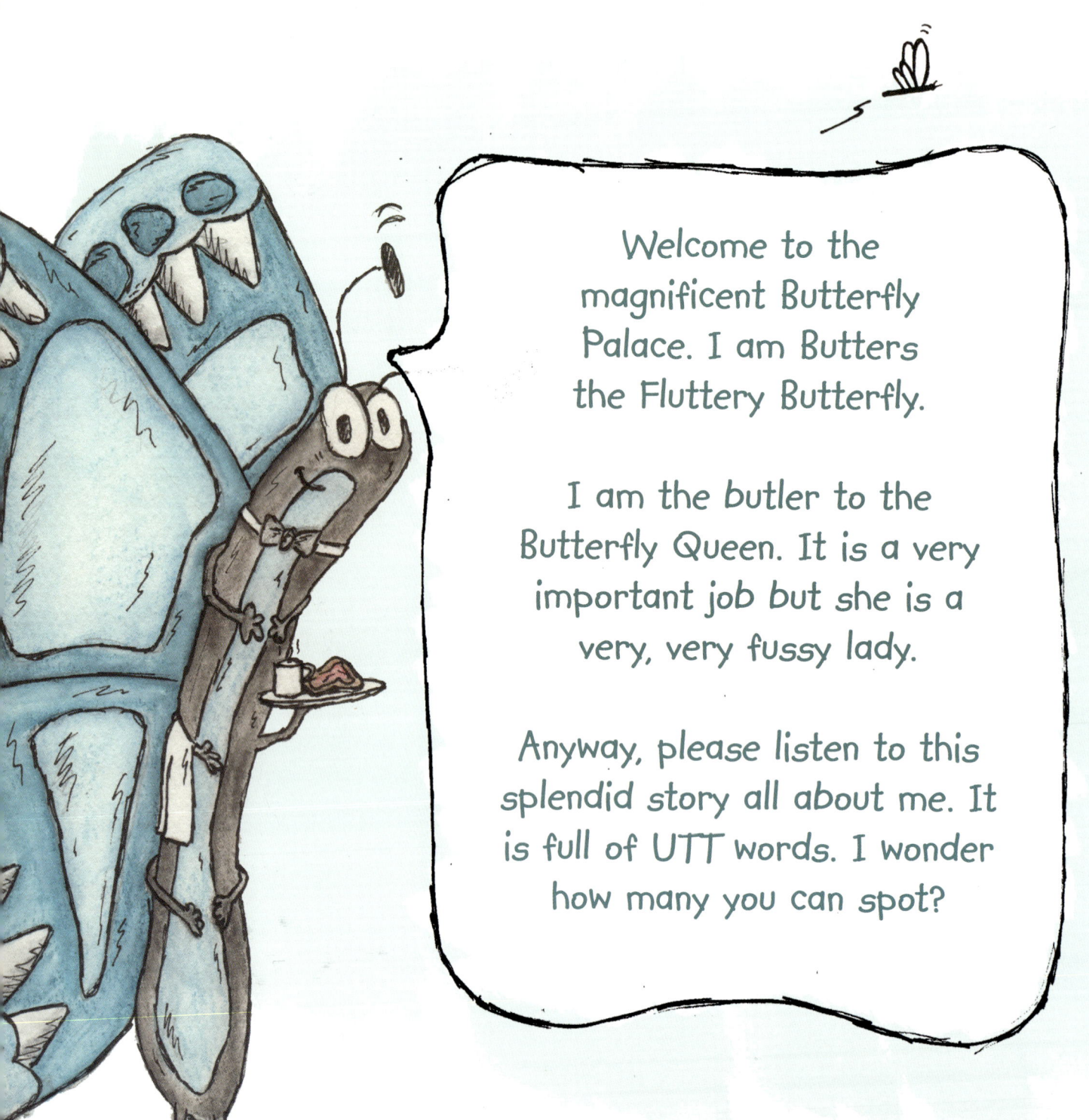

Welcome to the magnificent Butterfly Palace. I am Butters the Fluttery Butterfly.

I am the butler to the Butterfly Queen. It is a very important job but she is a very, very fussy lady.

Anyway, please listen to this splendid story all about me. It is full of UTT words. I wonder how many you can spot?

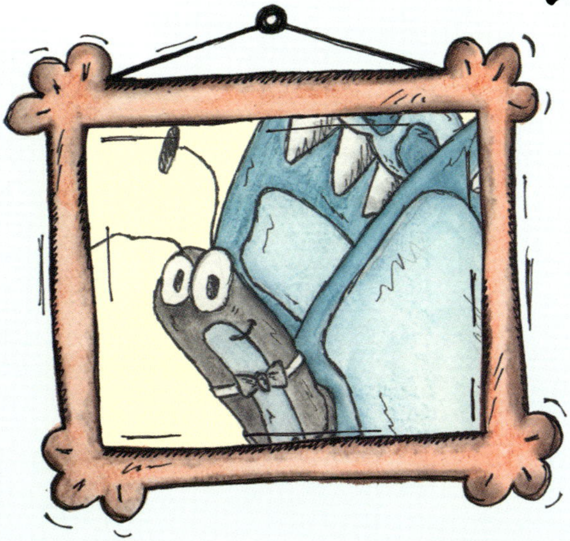

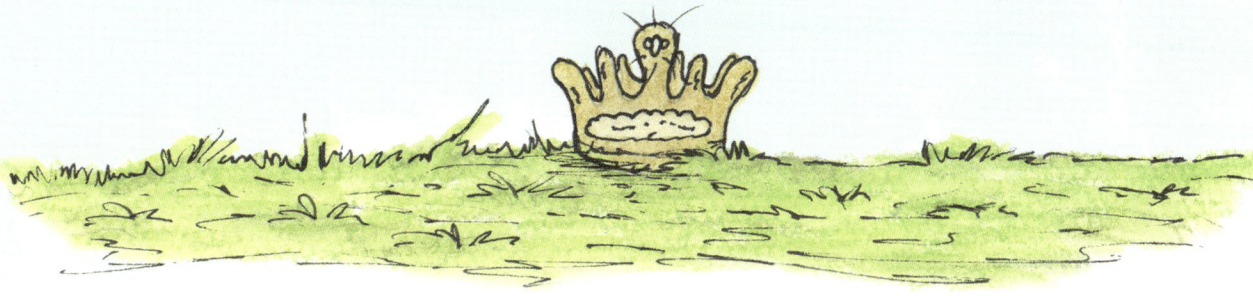

Butters the Fluttery Butterfly

Written by Craig Green and Dominic Vince
Illustrated by Sarah-Leigh Wills

Dear Anya.
Enjoy!
love Craig.
X.

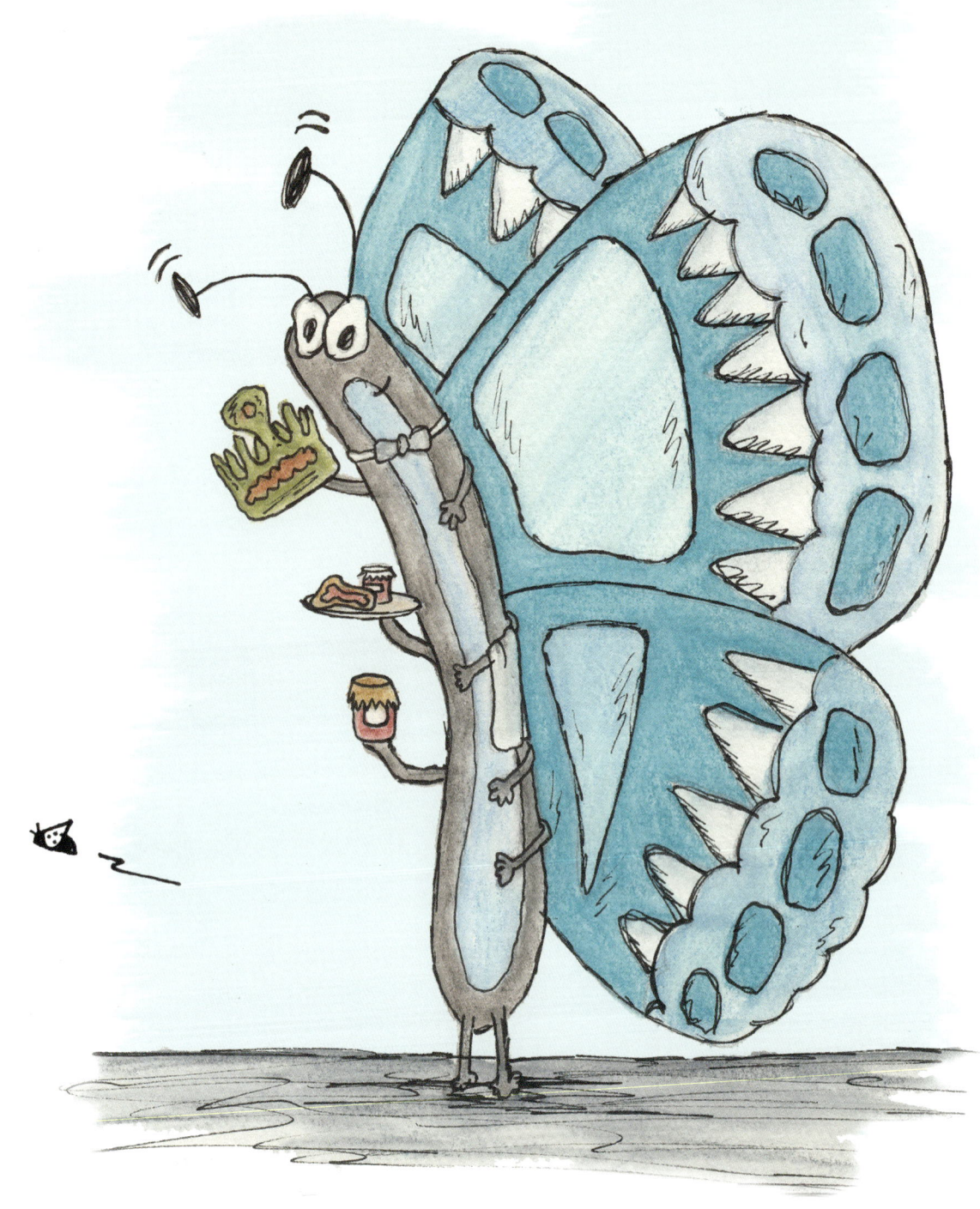

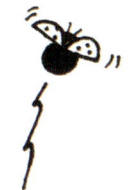

Butters the fluttery butterfly
Is a butler to the Queen,
He serves tea and buttered toast
With chutney, jam and cream.

Fluttery butterfly
fluttery butterfly
utt utt utt

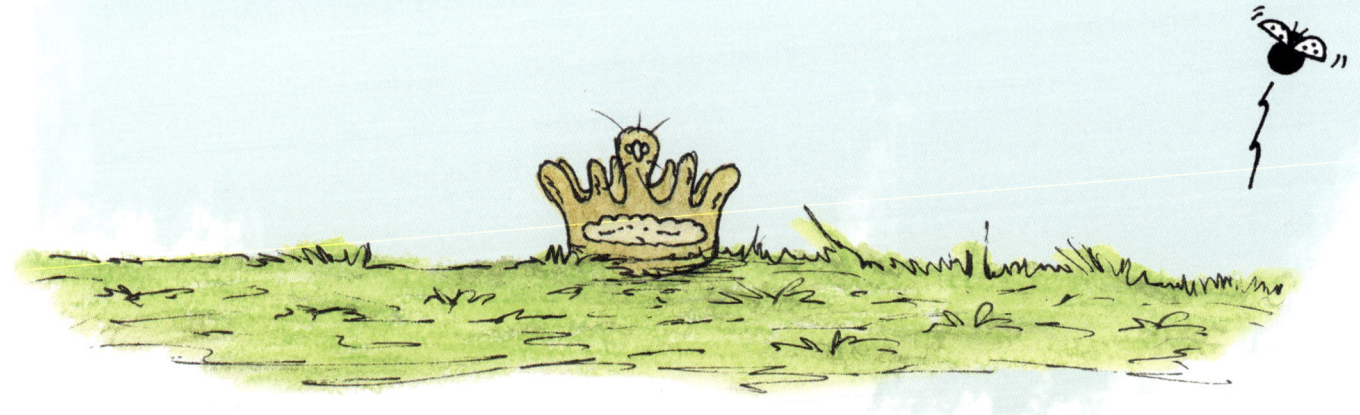

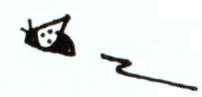

Fluttery butterfly
fluttery butterfly
UTT UTT UTT

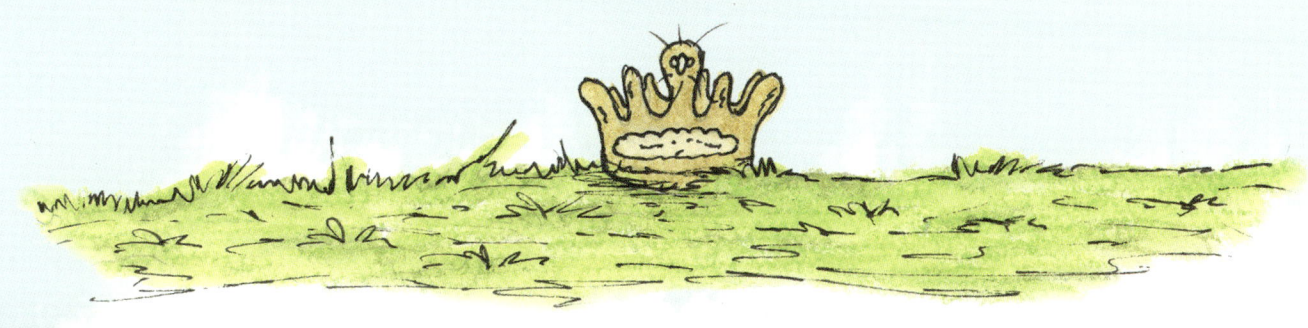

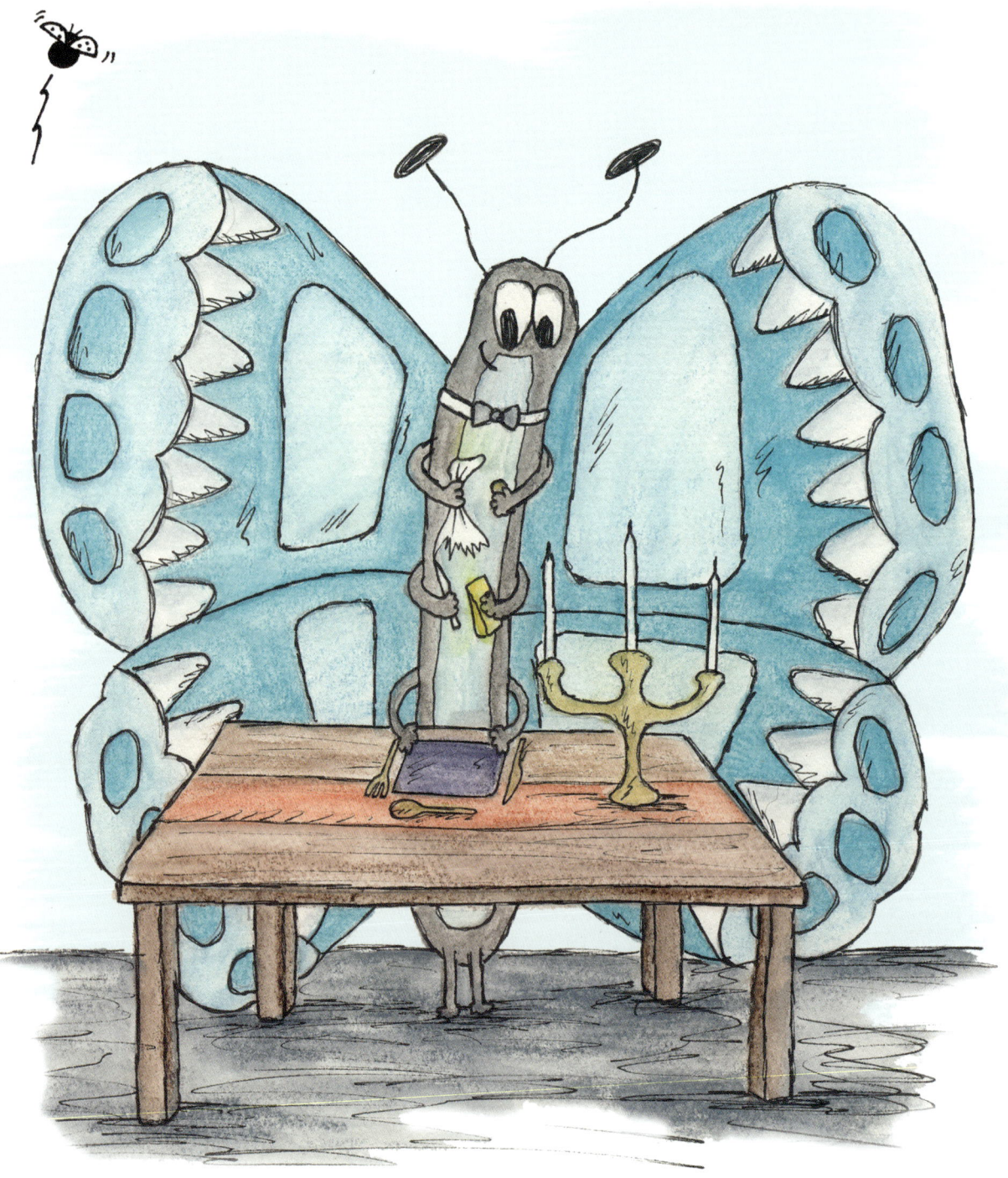

So utterly graceful is Butters
As he cuts the cheese and mutton,
And lays the cutlery and napkins
And shines the Queen's buttons.

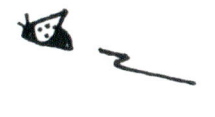

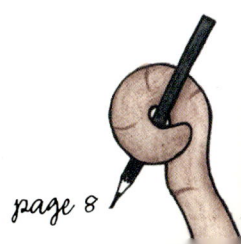

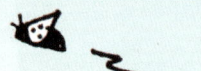

Fluttery butterfly
fluttery butterfly
utt utt utt

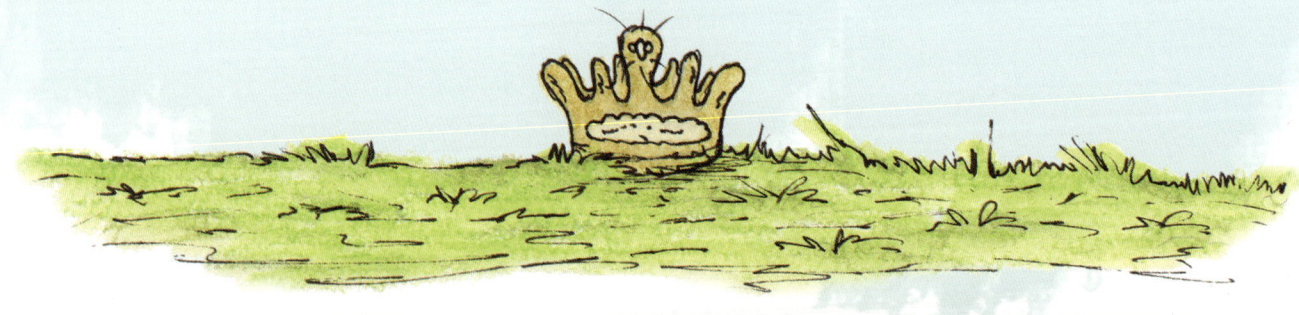

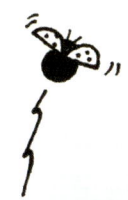

Fluttery butterfly
fluttery butterfly
UTT UTT UTT

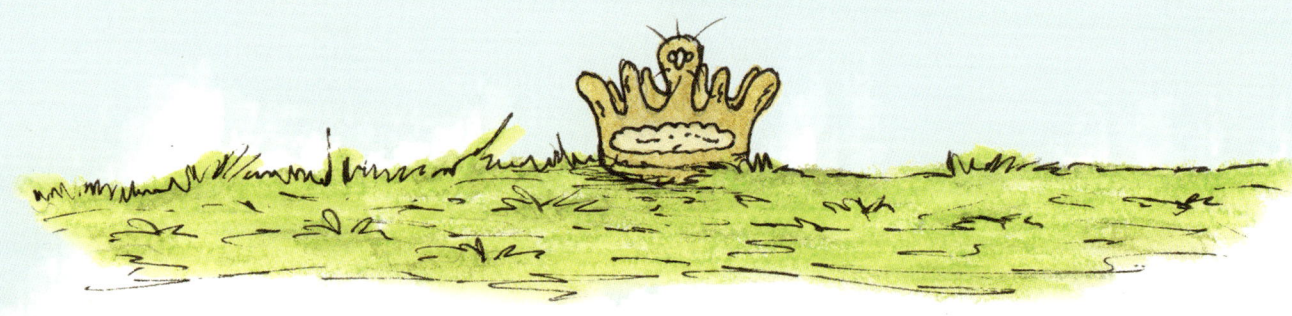

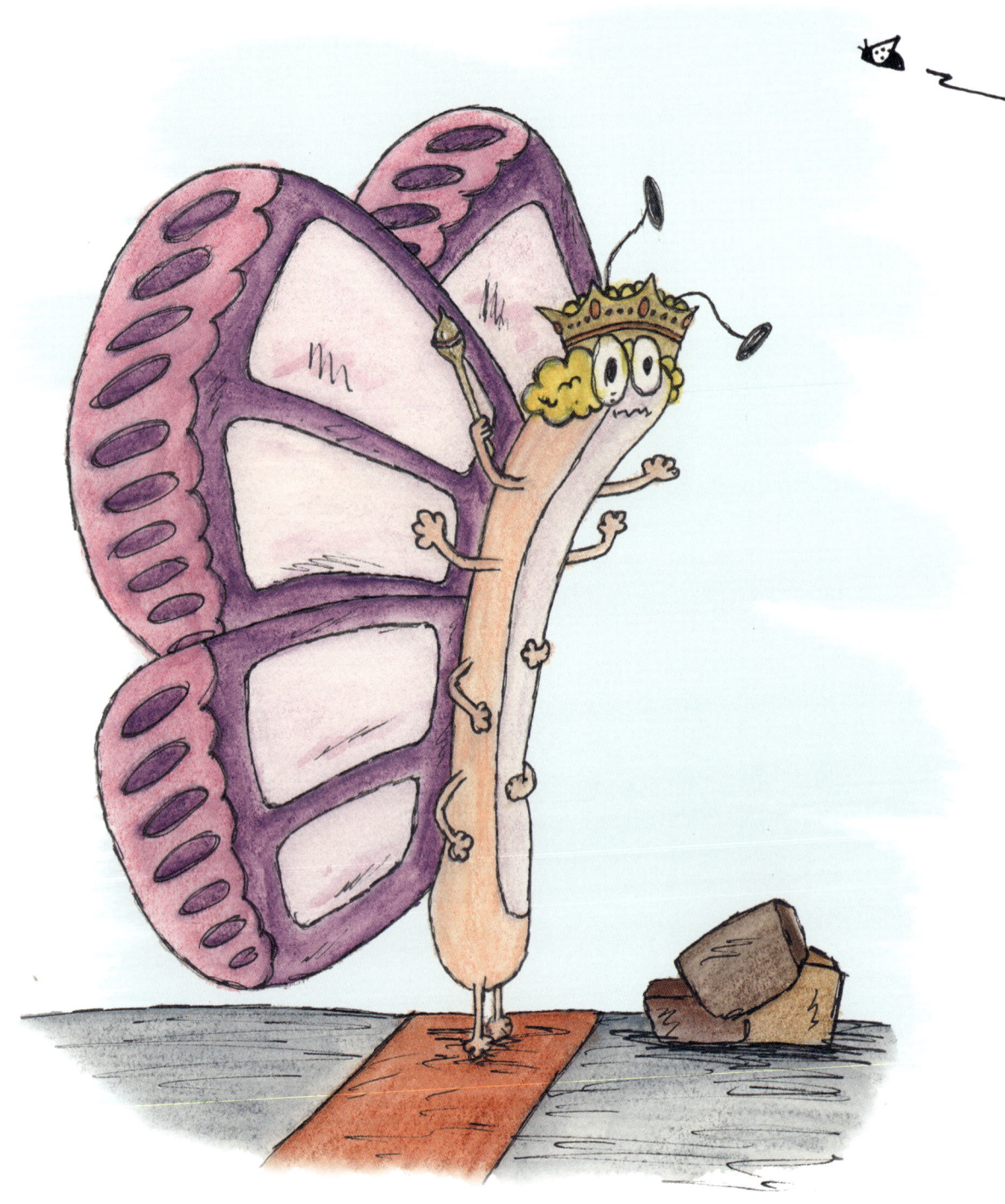

"Tut tut!" said the Queen one day,
"My palace is just so cluttered!"
And as she nuttily muttered
and spluttered,
Butters started to tidy away.

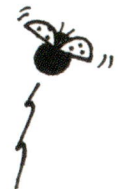

Fluttery butterfly
fluttery butterfly
utt utt utt

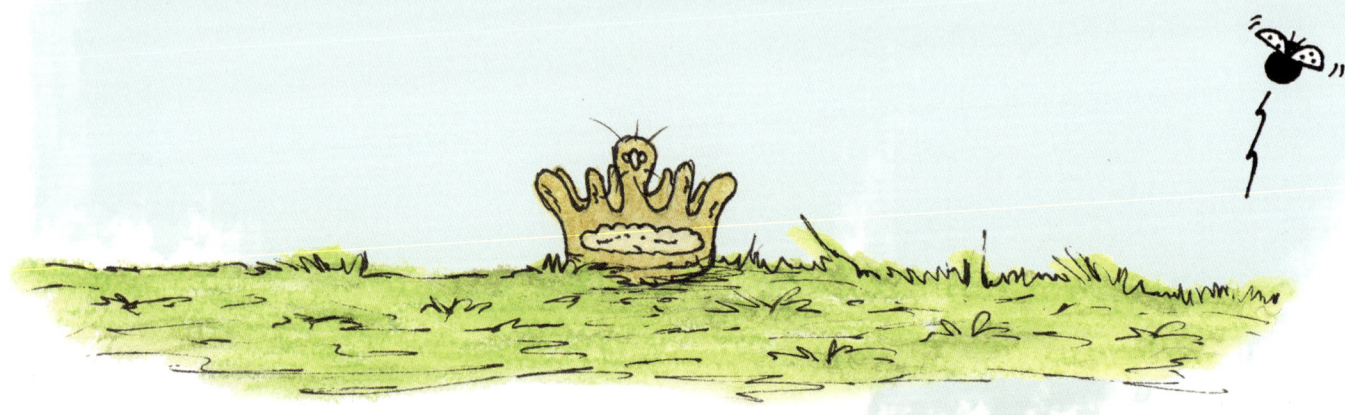

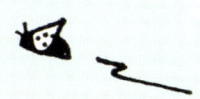

Fluttery butterfly
fluttery butterfly
UTT UTT UTT

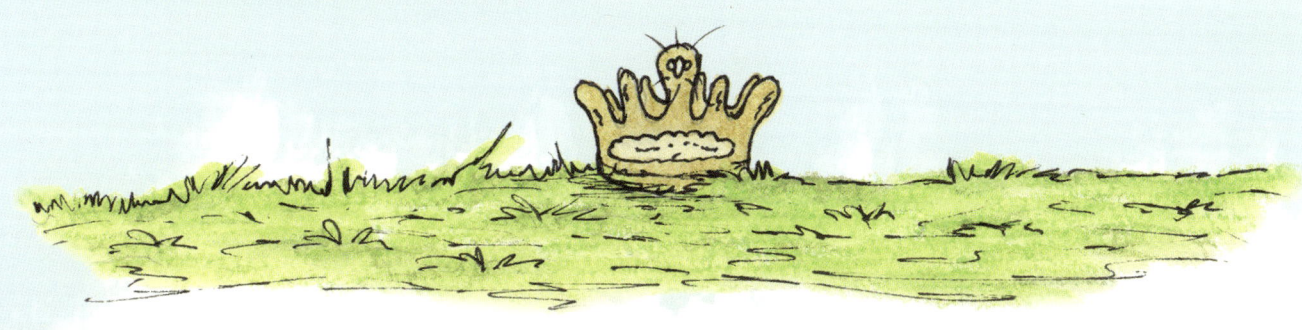

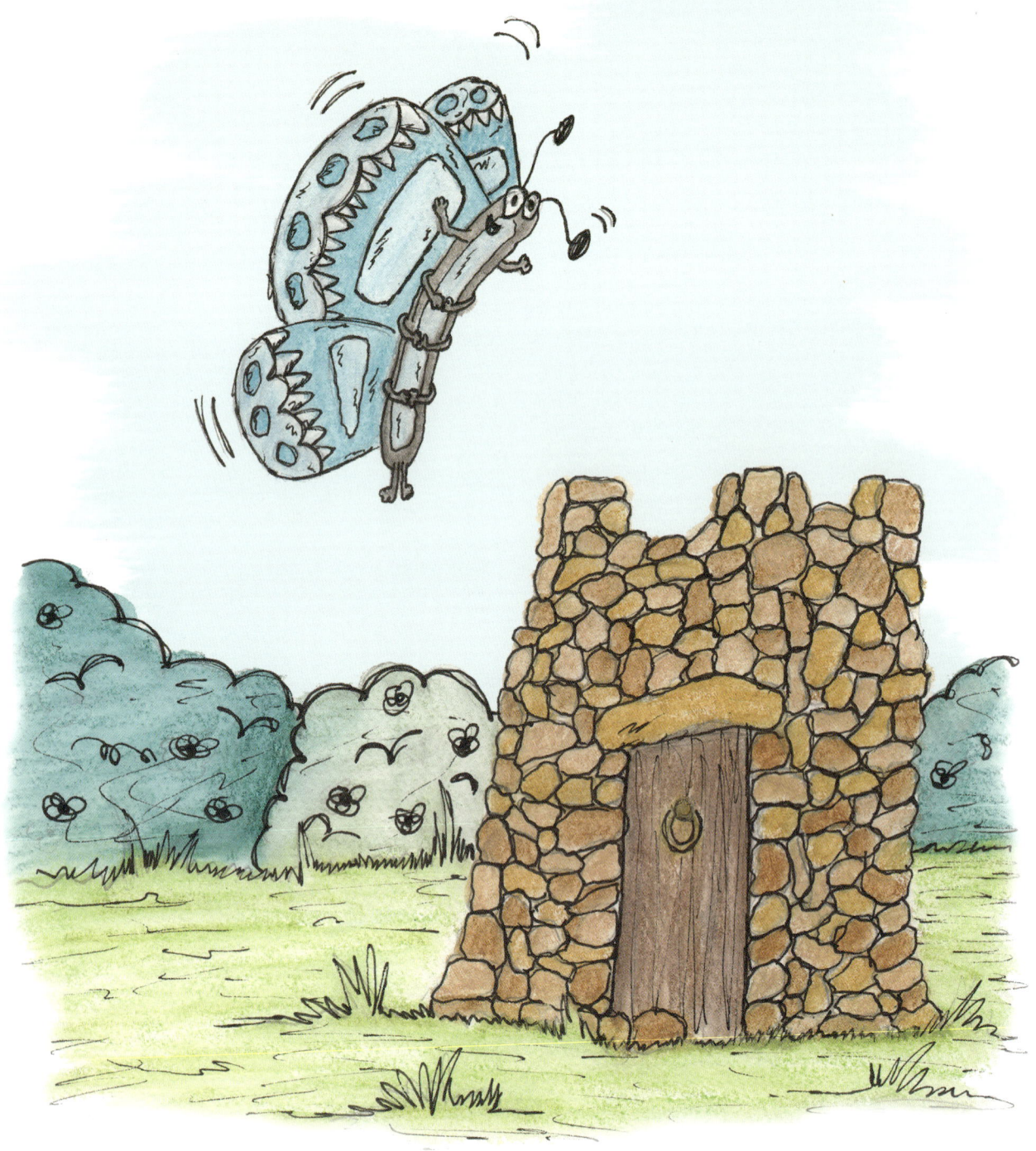

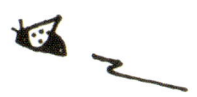

He fluttered about the palace
And shut all the clutter away
In a hut made of nuts in the garden,
And the Queen was happy all day.

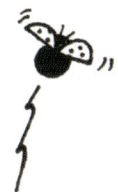

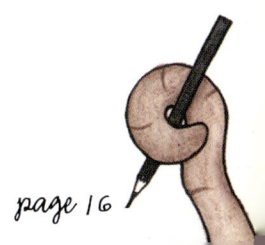

Fluttery butterfly
fluttery butterfly
utt utt utt

Fluttery butterfly
fluttery butterfly
UTT UTT UTT

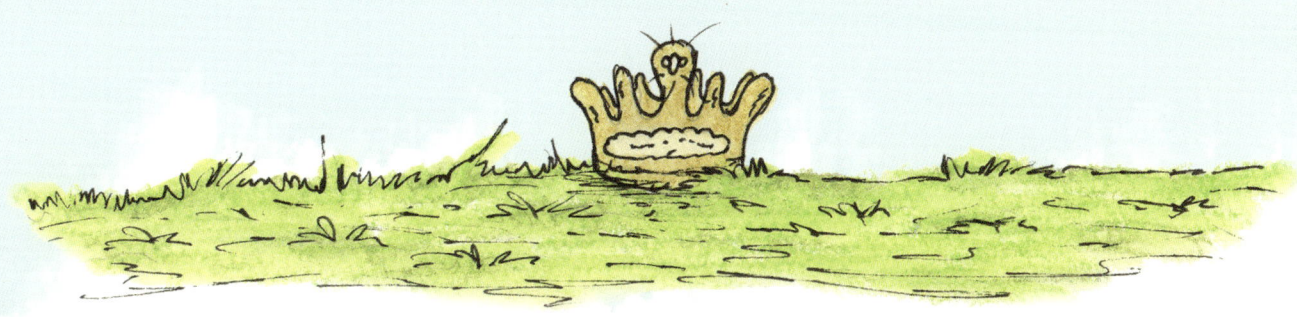

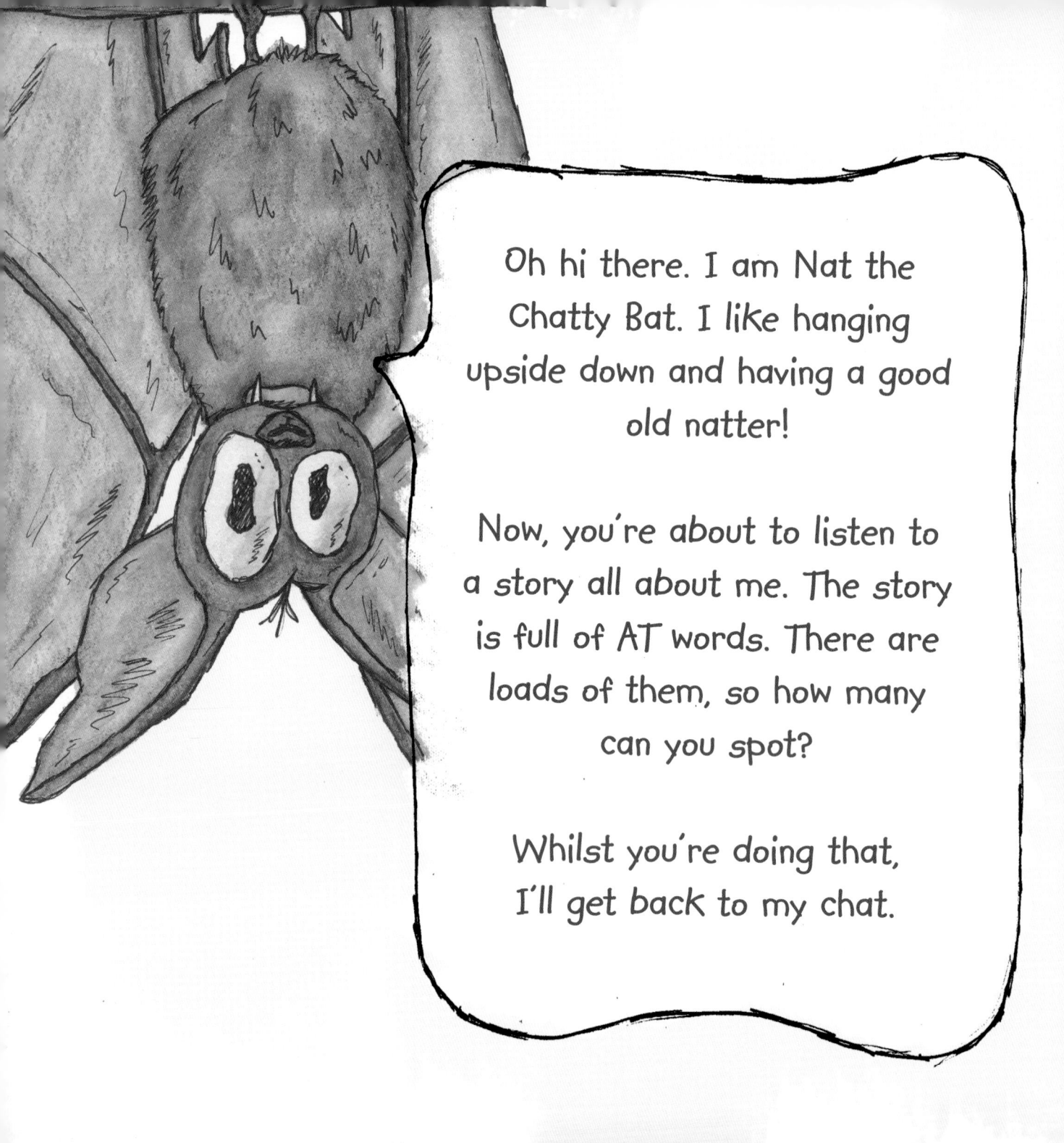

Oh hi there. I am Nat the Chatty Bat. I like hanging upside down and having a good old natter!

Now, you're about to listen to a story all about me. The story is full of AT words. There are loads of them, so how many can you spot?

Whilst you're doing that, I'll get back to my chat.

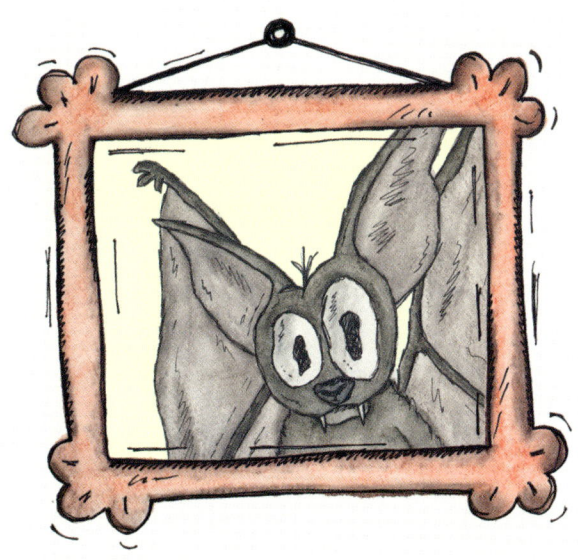

Nat the
Chatty Bat

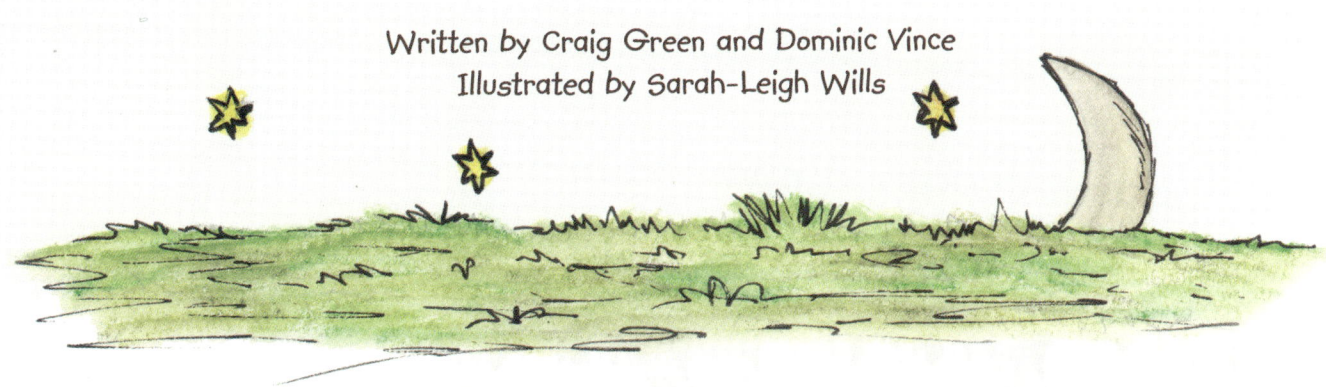

Written by Craig Green and Dominic Vince
Illustrated by Sarah-Leigh Wills

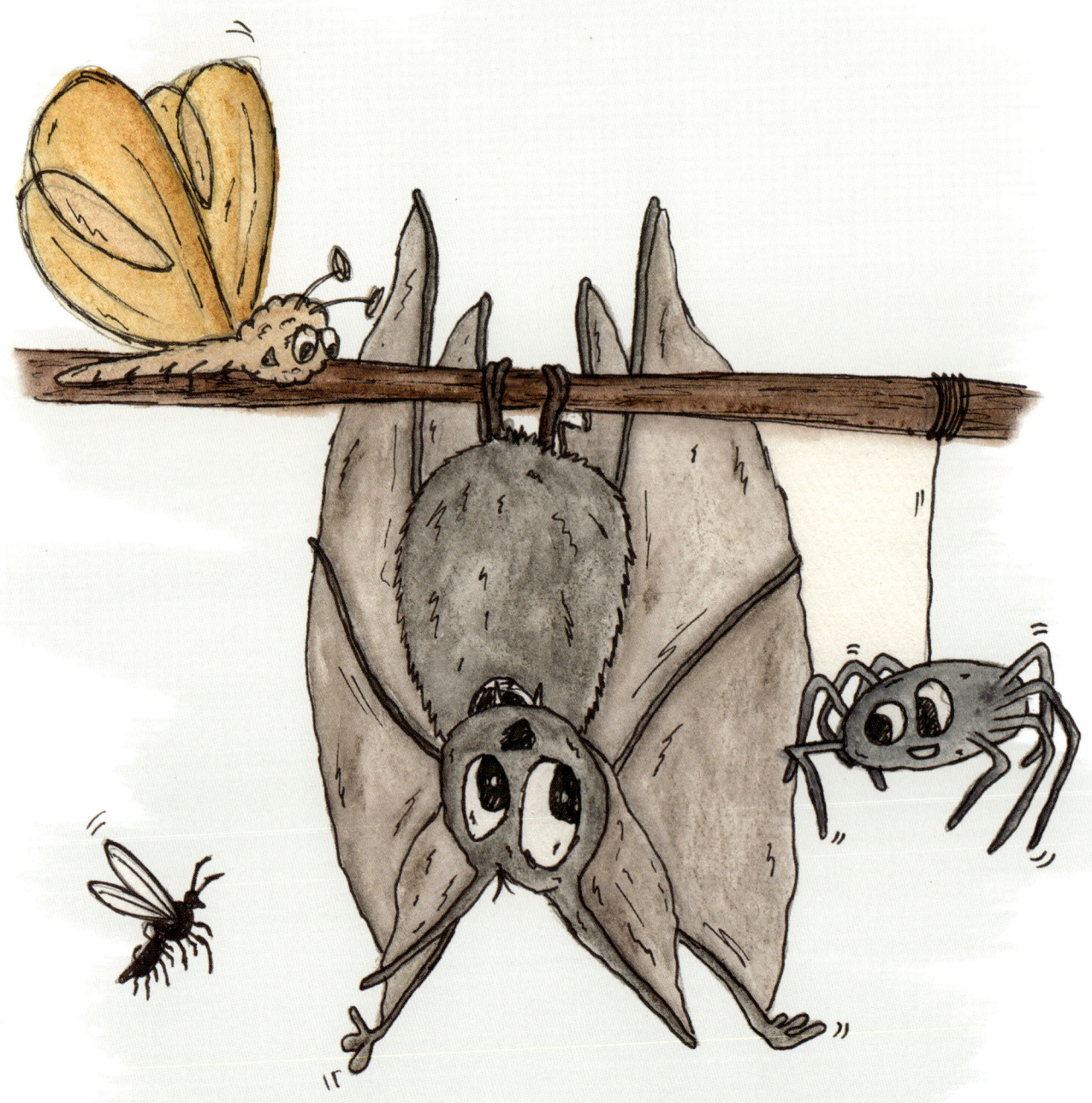

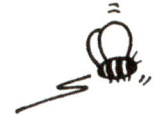

Nat the bat is small and fat
And loves to chitter, chatter, chat.
She chats to the horses, dogs and cats,
She chats to spiders, moths and gnats.

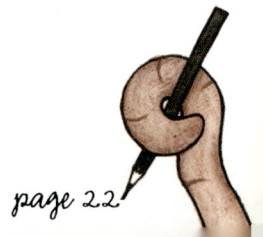

Chatty bat
chatty bat
at at at

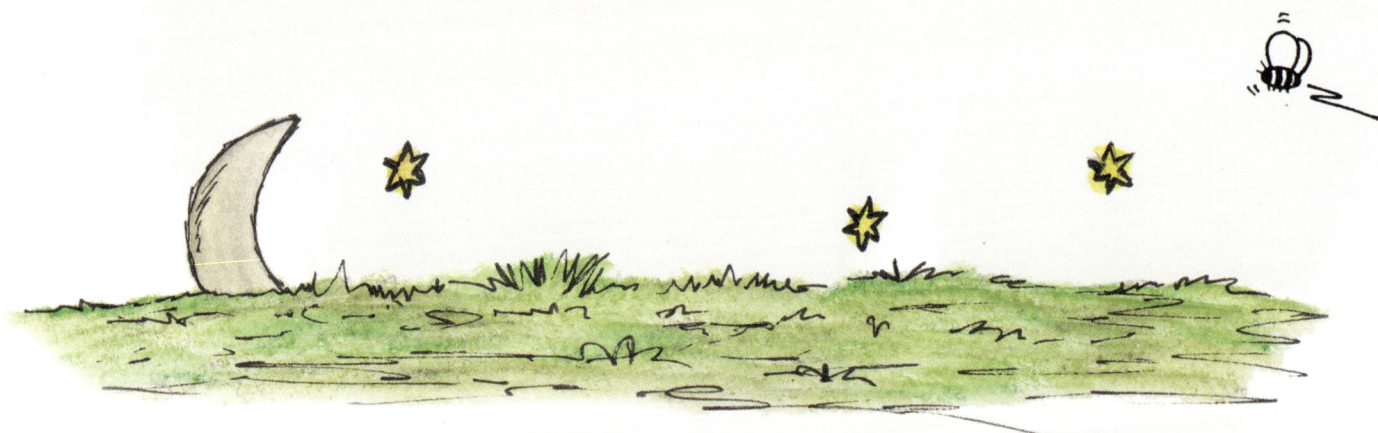

Chatty bat
chatty bat
AT AT AT

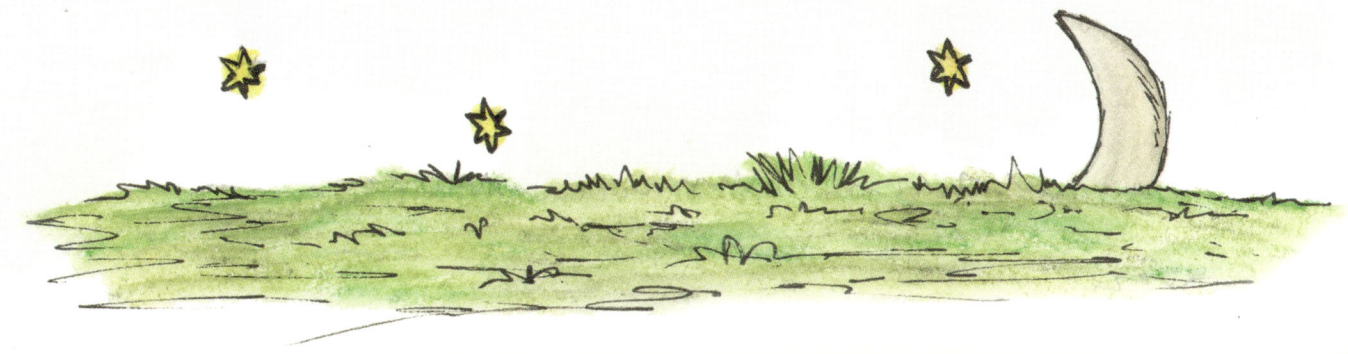

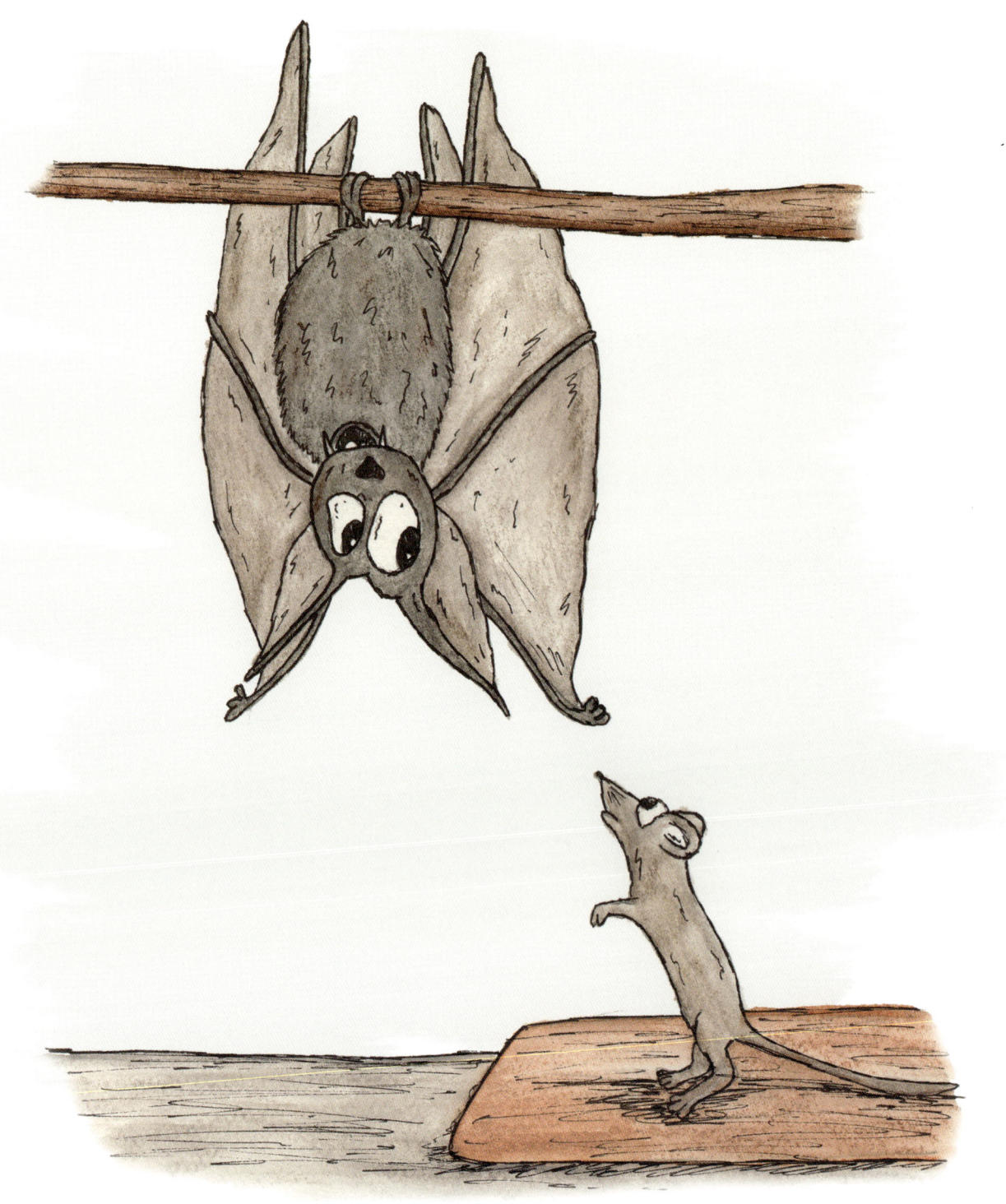

Pitter-patter on the mat,
Her friend the rat joins in the chat.
The problem is they chat all day,
The cats all wish they'd go away.

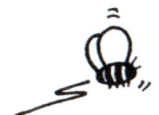

Chatty bat
chatty bat
at at at

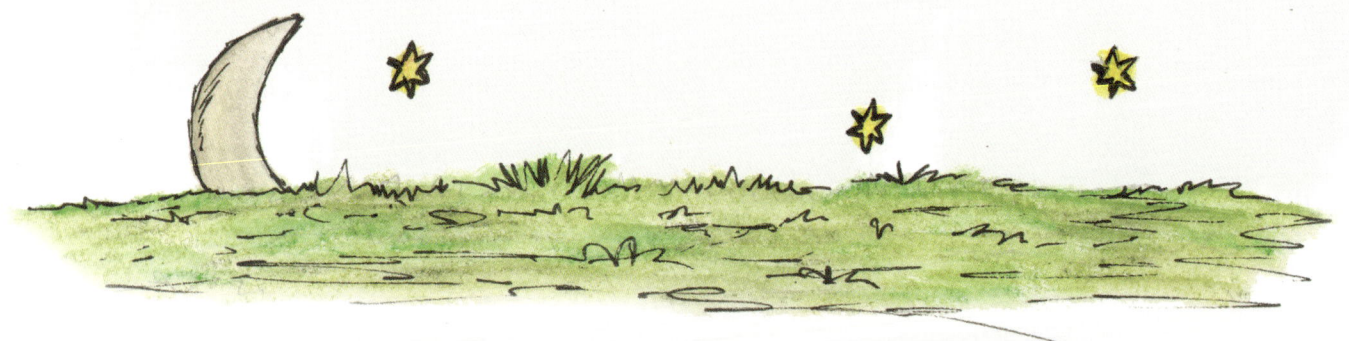

Chatty bat
chatty bat
AT AT AT

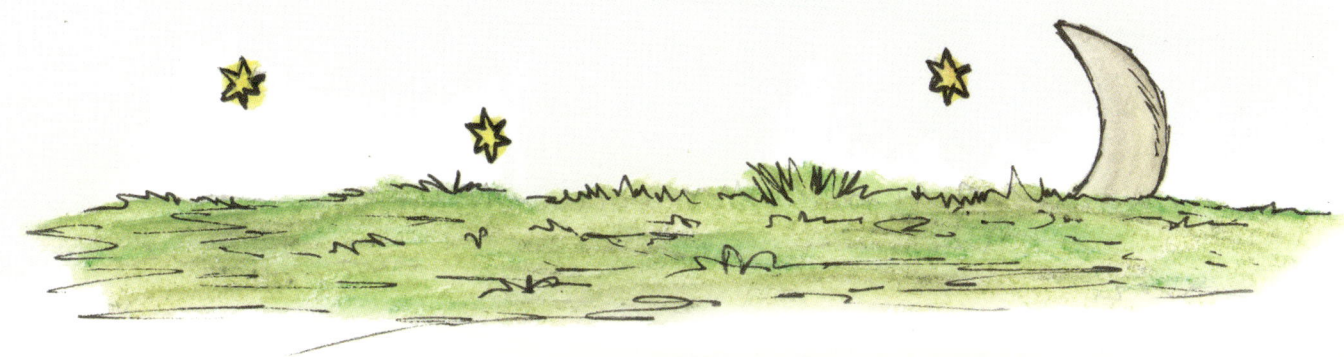

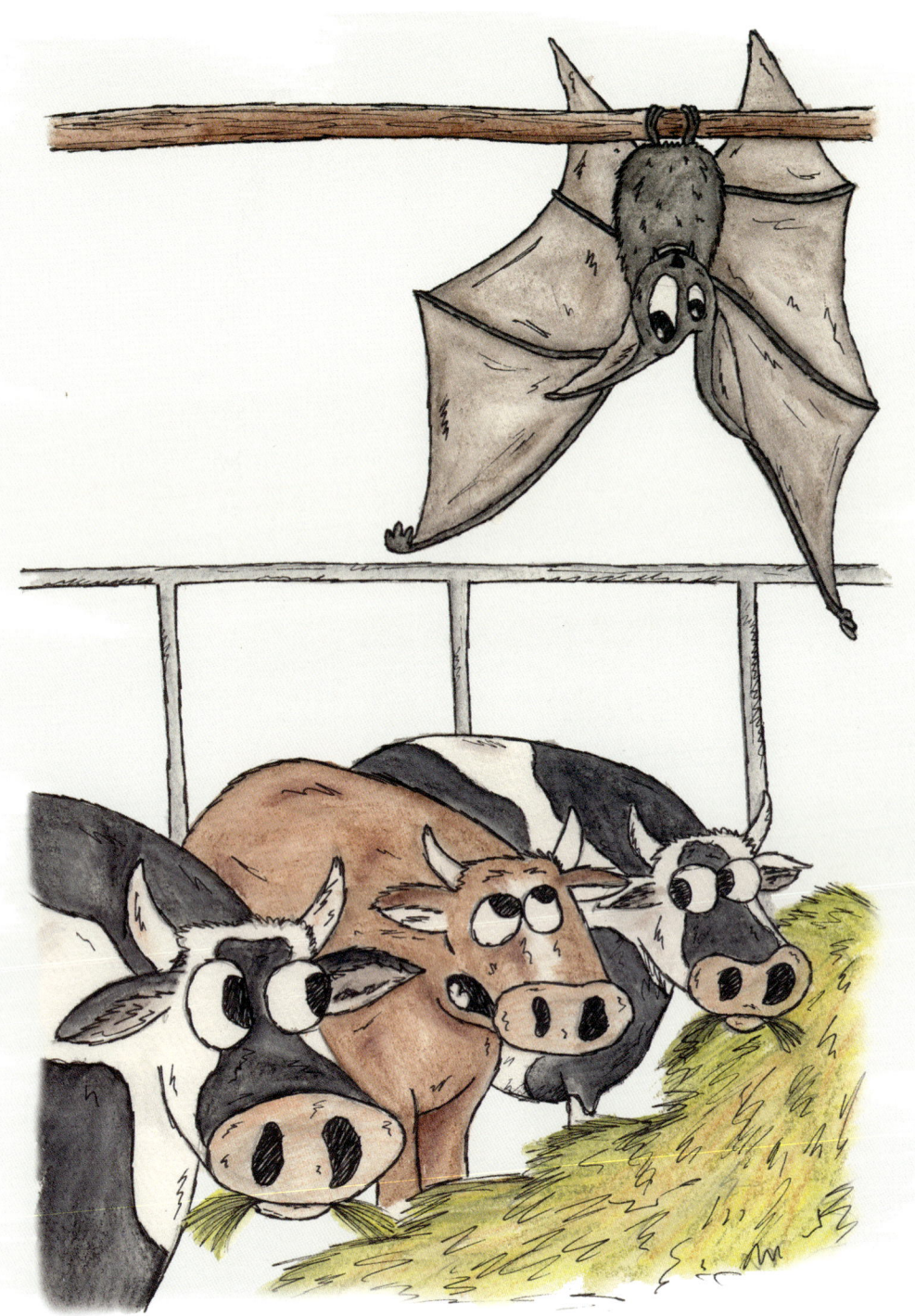

Nat lives above the dozing cattle
Way up in the attic high.
The cows can't bear the noisy prattle,
"Stop this chatter now!" they sigh.

Chatty bat
chatty bat
at at at

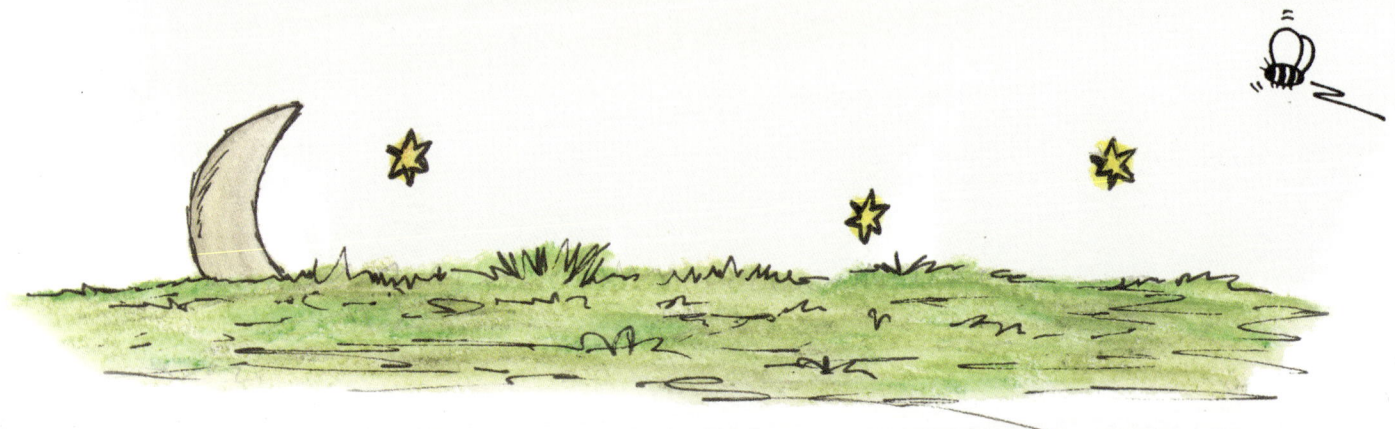

Chatty bat
chatty bat
AT AT AT

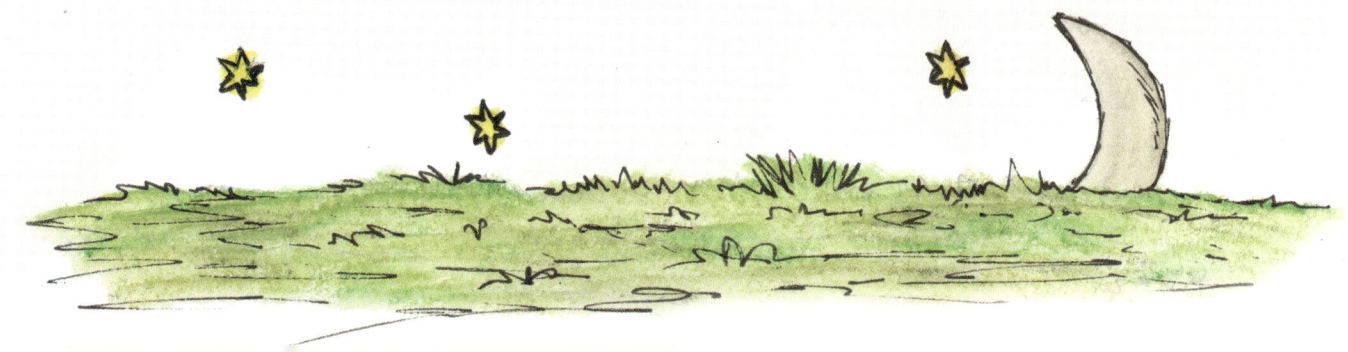

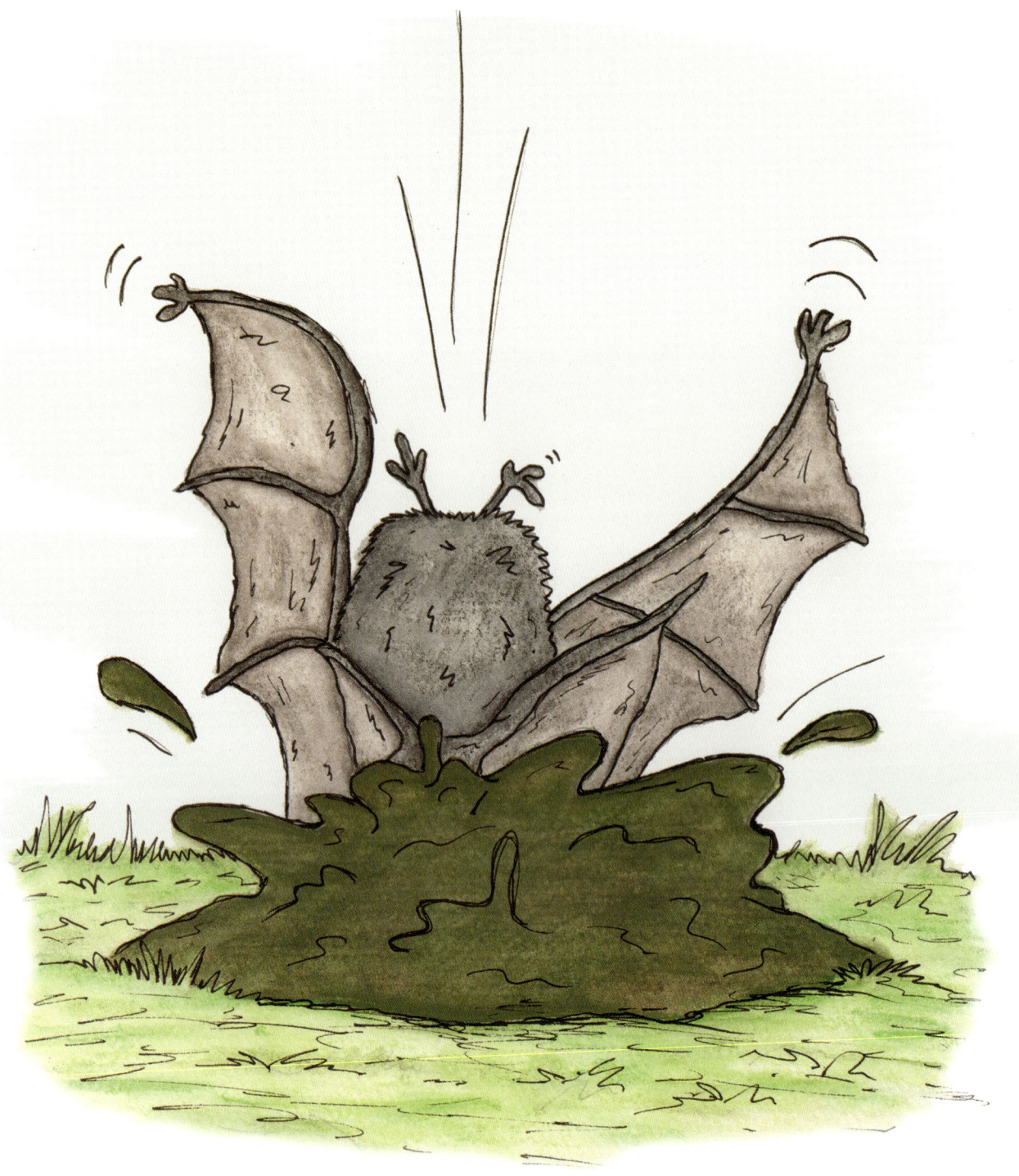

She likes to fly acrobatically
But one day fell dramatically
And landed flat with a mighty splat!
In a big green stinky cowpat!

Chatty bat
chatty bat
at at at

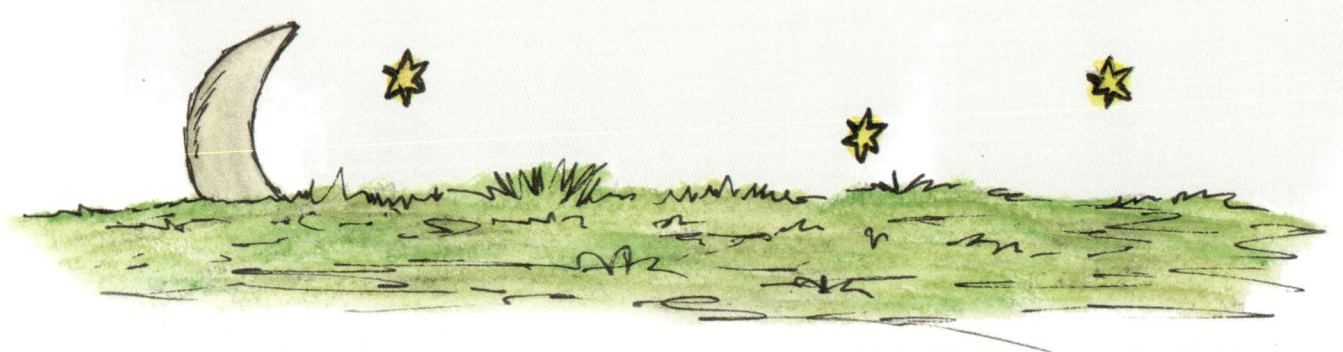

Chatty bat
chatty bat
AT AT AT

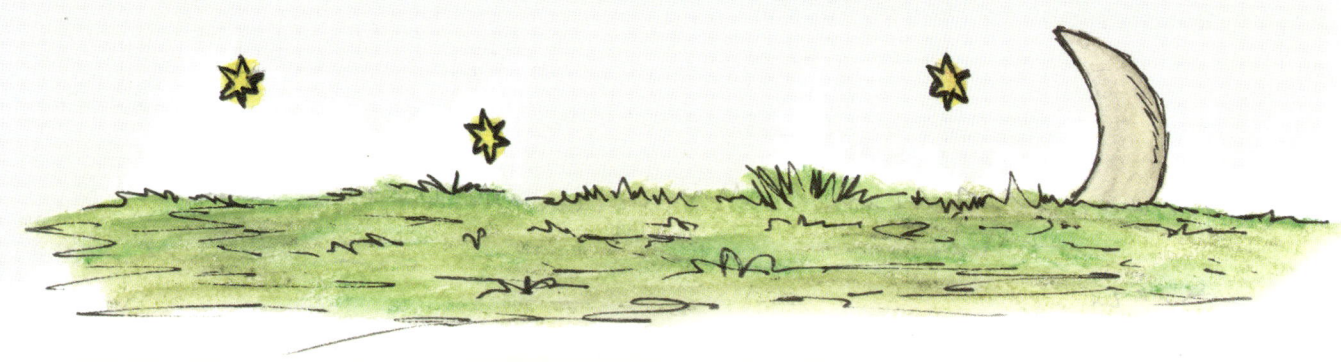

Your Clickety CD

This Clickety CD contains the two stories Butters the Fluttery Butterfly and Nat the Chatty Bat read by the amazing Catherine Tate.

You can listen or read along to the stories – listen carefully for the sound that tells you when to turn the page.

How many UTT and AT words can you spot?

CD produced by Matt Bernard and Jay Auborn at Deep Blue Sound.

Music written and produced by Jay Auborn.

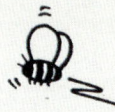

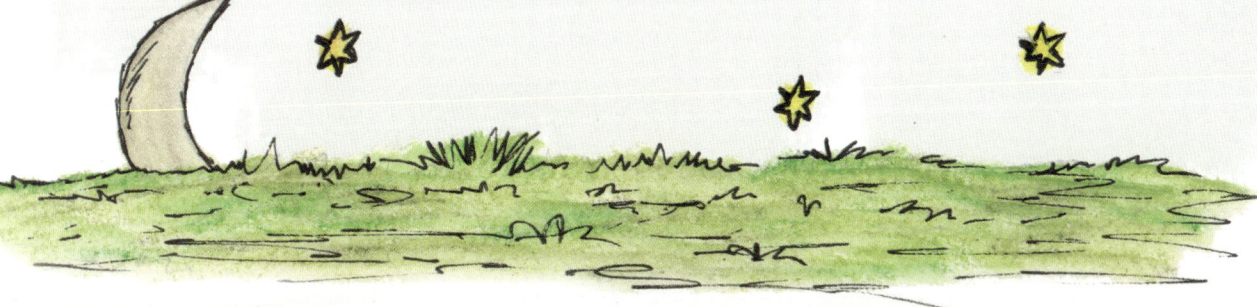